Praise for The *Opioid-Free Pain Relief Kit*

"A superb self-help book that uses cognitive-beha[vioral] recovery from chronic pain. Easy to read and to [use,] and focused text will provide both the informati[on that] chronic pain sufferers can utilize to restore normal activities."

— *John Loeser, MD, Professor, University of Washington*
Past President, American Pain Society and
the International Association for the Study of Pain

"Pain, fear of pain, and pain pills form a vicious cycle. This book, written by a real expert, can help you break the cycle. Small, doable steps lead away from pills, lessen the pain, and diminish much of the fear. All this leads to a fuller, more productive and more joyful life. Go for it! You have nothing to lose but your pain, and so much to gain."

— *Kate Lorig, DrPH, director and professor emeritus, Stanford*
University School of Medicine's Patient Education Research Center

"This book provides a comprehensive and accessible guide that will inspire and empower those with chronic pain to take back their lives, without relying on dangerous medications. It is a must read for those living with pain."

— *Jennifer L. Murphy, PhD, VA CBT for Chronic Pain Trainer,*
Clinical Director, Chronic Pain Rehabilitation Program, James A.
Haley Veterans' Hospital, Tampa, Florida

"Patients are looking for options now that opioids have been found to be less effective than once thought. Alternative approaches are frequently suggested but with little guidance on where to seek help. *The Opioid-Free Pain Relief Kit* is an excellent, patient centered, practical approach to taking back control over pain that often ruins the lives of our patients. With Beth's Tips and patient scenarios, the text is interesting and informative. Enjoyable graphics and forms to guide progress makes the book a discovery and not a chore. This volume begs for our patients to enlist their time and energy and for us to review their success, a refreshing addition to the patient's own resource guide."

— *Bill McCarberg, MD, Immediate Past President,*
American Academy of Pain Medicine

"The latest book by Dr. Darnall gives individuals with chronic pain a practical, step-by-step approach to reduce pain and become less reliant on pain medications"

> —W. Michael Hooten, MD, Division of Pain Medicine, Mayo Clinic,
> Rochester, Minnesota

"*The Opioid-Free Pain Relief Kit* is a workbook for people with chronic pain and in my mind it is an instant classic. Dr. Darnall clearly and gently explains the basic principles of chronic pain and how people can help themselves. Pain patients have for too long felt totally dependent on healthcare providers for pain relief: *"Who will help me?" "What will they do to help me?"* and *"What am I going to be prescribed?"* This book explains how pain patients have the ability to significantly decrease their pain and take charge of their own pain relief. I will be recommending this book to all of my patients."

> —Ted Jones, PhD, Lead Psychologist, Pain Consultants of
> East Tennessee

"A straightforward, easy-to-read book containing the key ingredients necessary for anyone to develop their own plan for managing chronic pain."

> —Steven Dobscha, MD, Professor, Department of Psychiatry,
> Oregon Health & Science University

"Dr. Beth Darnall has again provided a highly-readable, practical, understandable and insightful guide for the chronic pain sufferer. It is a wonderful adjunct and standalone book that can truly make a difference leading to less suffering, increased function, and a happier life. I recommend it highly to medical care professionals and individuals with chronic pain conditions. Reading this book will result in a positive life-changing experience."

> —Steven D. Feinberg, MD, MPH,
> Board Certified, Physical Medicine & Rehabilitation
> Board Certified, American Board of Pain Medicine
> Past-President of the American Academy of Pain Medicine

The Opioid-Free Pain Relief Kit

10 Simple Steps to Ease Your Pain

Beth Darnall, PhD

Features:

- ❖ Relaxation Recording to Calm Your Nervous System
- ❖ Easy-to-Use Pain Psychology Skills
- ❖ Your Plan for Pain Relief
- ❖ Opioid Education

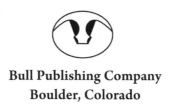

Bull Publishing Company
Boulder, Colorado

Published by Bull Publishing Company
P.O. Box 1377
Boulder, CO, USA 80306
www.bullpub.com

Library of Congress Cataloging-in-Publication Data
Names: Darnall, Beth, author.
Title: The opioid-free pain relief kit : 10 simple steps to ease your pain /
    by Beth Darnall, PhD.
Description: Boulder, Colorado : Bull Publishing Company, [2016] |
    Includes bibliographical references and index.
Identifiers: LCCN 2016022357 | ISBN 978-1-936693-98-6 (softbound :
    alk. paper) |
Subjects: LCSH: Chronic pain--Alternative treatment--Popular works. |
    Chronic pain--Psychological aspects--Popular works. | Mind and body
    therapies--Popular works. | Self-care, Health--Popular works.
Classification: LCC RB127 .D393 2016 | DDC 616/.0472--dc23
LC record available at https://lccn.loc.gov/2016022357

Printed in USA

22 21 20 19 18   10 9 8 7 6 5 4 3

Interior design and project management: Dovetail Publishing Services
Cover design and production: Shannon Bodie, Lightbourne, Inc.

Contents

Acknowledgments

My heartfelt gratitude to Sean Mackey, MD, PhD for your enduring support, and to Nita Bryant and my incredible publishing team: Jim Bull and Erin Mulligan, Claire Cameron, Emily Sewell, and Jon Peck; this was a lightning speed team effort and I am blessed to work with all of you.

I hold deep respect for the clinicians who work tirelessly on the front lines each day to help others have less pain. My hope is that this book serves as a valuable clinical resource for you and those you serve. To the millions who are living with pain and are searching for ways to help themselves suffer less: The power to change your experience and your life is inside you, waiting to be unlocked. This book stands as my collective message of hope to you, and in these pages you will find keys. Finally, I hold gratitude for my past chronic pain because suffering was an invaluable teacher that served to shape my message and my mission.

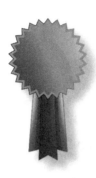

CONGRATULATIONS!

Picking up this book shows you want to help yourself feel better. That's the first step toward having less pain and using less pain medication.

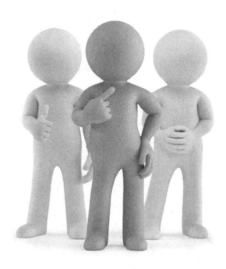

You are not alone. About 100 million Americans—one in three people—have ongoing pain. Health professionals refer to pain that is ongoing as **chronic pain.** Chronic pain is defined as pain that lasts longer than 6 months. It can be mild or very strong, come in waves or always be present, be simply annoying or make your normal life hard to live. Pain is the most common reason people visit their doctor. Many people mistakenly believe that chronic pain is best treated simply by taking powerful

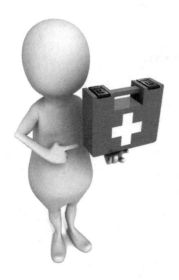

painkillers, also known as opioids.* But people who think pills are the only answer are mistaken, because the best treatment for chronic pain includes much more than pills.

In fact, the most important part of pain treatment isn't your medication or even your doctor: it's YOU. This book gives you the right road map and skills to help you reduce your own pain, so you need less medication. It is a formula for success—your own personal pain relief kit.

---

*A few examples of brand-name opioid painkillers include Oxycontin, Percocet, Vicodin, and Norco. To learn more about opioid medications, see page 107

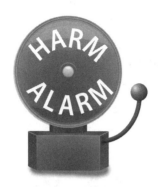

STEP 1
Quiet Your "Harm Alarm"

Pain is your "HARM ALARM"

Pain grabs your attention. And, because it is so unpleasant, pain motivates you to escape whatever is causing it. The pain you feel after placing your hand on a hot stove will make you quickly move your hand away from the burner, thereby preventing further injury.

Just like a fire alarm warning you of danger, pain usually signals a threat. **Humans are born with the natural instinct to escape pain and threats, and seek safety.** After all, escaping threats is what helped us to evolve and survive as a species. Pain sounds the "Harm Alarm", and your brain and your body work together to prepare you for a fast getaway. Your nervous system goes on high alert and triggers changes that help you escape whatever is *causing* pain—such as the hot stove.

Here's how your nervous system prepares you to escape the cause of your pain:

 Your muscles tense.

 Your breathing speeds up.

 Your heartbeat speeds up.

 Your blood vessels constrict.

 Fight-or-flight chemicals are released into your blood.

You may notice some of these changes in your body, such as muscle tension and quick breathing, when you are facing or experiencing ordinary pain, but they usually go away after the cause of the pain is gone. With chronic pain, however, these changes happen continuously in your nervous system. As a result, you may become so used to these changes that you no longer notice they are happening—especially if you are more focused on your pain. And, over time, these changes just become "the new normal," meaning that your muscles are always tight and your breathing is always quick and shallow.

These changes are meant to help you "escape" pain—to help you run from a hungry tiger or pull your hand away from the stove, for example. But you cannot escape chronic pain by running

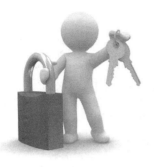 away or hiding. After all, how do you escape pain when it's coming from inside you? Because we evolved to flee pain, having no clear action to take in the case of chronic pain can be confusing and distressing. Given how humans are wired, it's no wonder that chronic pain can cause stress and anxiety. It can also lead to feelings of helplessness and depression.

Calming Your Nervous System and Quieting Your "Harm Alarm"

Having your nervous system on high alert all the time is not helpful and actually makes your chronic pain worse. **A key part of chronic pain relief involves calming your nervous system—and quieting your "Harm Alarm."**

Wanting quick relief is natural, and that is why taking opioid medication can *seem* like a good solution. But it is better to calm your nervous system and quiet your "Harm Alarm" naturally using simple skills. These skills can provide a big part of the pain relief the pills provide—without all the side effects and risks!

Nervous System on High Alert ⟶ More Pain

Calm Nervous System ⟶ Pain Relief

Using the Pain Relief Recording to Quiet your "Harm Alarm"

Your pain relief recording is an audio file designed to quiet your "Harm Alarm." Listening to the recording will calm your nervous system. It guides you to slow your breathing, and you learn how to breathe from your diaphragm—so-called deep "belly" breathing, or *diaphragmatic breathing.* It's important to work with your breath because it helps dampen pain processing in your nervous system. Diaphragmatic breathing signals to your brain that it's safe to settle into a deep state of relaxation.

Other positive changes will soon follow your slowed breathing: your heartbeat will slow, your muscles will relax, and your mind will calm. It's your antidote to your "Harm Alarm"! As you listen, you will notice differences in your breathing and muscles right away. Listen to the recording regularly and you will do more than just feel better in the moment—you will train your brain away from pain.

How to Use the Pain Relief Recording to Calm Your Nervous System and Quiet Your "Harm Alarm"

1. On a computer or other device, **locate the relaxation recording** that comes with this book at www.bullpub.com /catalog/EPM.

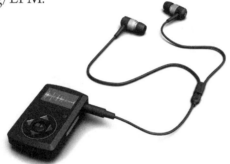

2. For the first few weeks, **set aside 20 minutes a day** to devote your full attention to the recording.

3. **Find a quiet space** where you can get into a comfortable position and close your eyes.

4. Before you listen to the recording, **take stock of how you feel.** Use the Stress Scale on page 8 to rate your overall level of stress. Consider how much pain you are feeling at the moment, as well as any other things in your life that are causing you stress. Rate and write down your current stress level each time you sit down to listen to the recording. You can keep a record of your stress levels using the worksheet on page 16.

Rate your overall stress level on a scale from 0 to 10.

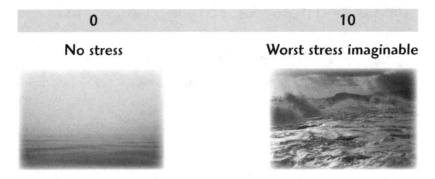

0	10
No stress	**Worst stress imaginable**

Your PRE-Treatment Stress Level: _____

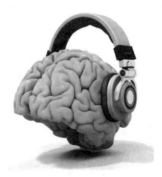

5. **Use headphones** to listen to the recording. The audio
   file contains *binaural technology* that works directly on
   your nervous system to help you settle into a deep state of
   relaxation. This advanced technology only works if you use
   headphones to listen to the recording.

6. Right after listening to the recording, **rate your stress level again** on a scale from 0 to 10.

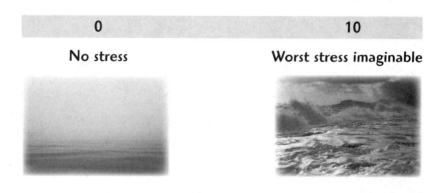

0	10
No stress	**Worst stress imaginable**

Your POST-Treatment Stress Level: _____

Did your stress level change after you listened to the recording?

Most people notice that their stress level has dropped after listening to the recording. Some people also notice that they have less pain. Use the worksheet on page 16 to keep track of your stress level before and after you listen to the recording, as well as any thoughts you may have about your progress.

Don't worry if you did not notice changes in your pain right away. Remember, pain causes your nervous system to be on high alert. And having your nervous system on high alert makes your chronic pain worse.

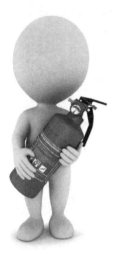

The goal of the recording is to calm your nervous system and quiet your "Harm Alarm." By calming your nervous system, your brain and body are no longer "primed" for future pain and an "escape" response. When you listen to the recording, you relax and teach your body that it's OK to be right where you are, in a state of deep relaxation. **Deep relaxation is the opposite of pain—it's your antidote!**

When you practice relaxation skills, your brain and body become less reactive to pain over time. In turn, this reduces your pain. It is normal for this to take a little while before you feel less pain. At first, just focus on using the recording regularly, with a goal of calming your nervous system. Trust that your pain will diminish if you listen to the recording regularly over time. Just like medication, it can take a few weeks to build up in your system to the point where you notice big changes in your pain.

Calming your nervous system daily will gain you relief. Used regularly, your brain and body will become less reactive and your pain will stay lower.

How often should I listen to the recording?

Listen to the recording at least once daily. Two or three times a day is even better!

Think of the recording as being mind-body medicine for your nervous system. It teaches you how to calm your thoughts so that your mind and body relax and feel less pain. These are important mind-body skills! Every time you listen to the recording, you are giving your nervous system a "dose" of calming medicine— medicine that counteracts pain by quieting the "Harm Alarm." Spread out your "doses" throughout the day to keep yourself in a calm, relaxed state that keeps your pain at bay.

Twenty minutes may seem like a lot of time, but it is an excellent investment. The goal is to train your brain away from pain, and this takes a little while. Remind yourself how much time your pain has taken away from you—and use that as motivation to invest in reclaiming it.

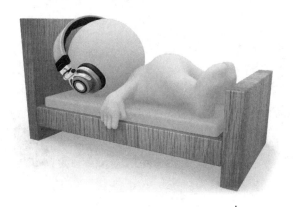

Can the recording help me sleep better?

Yes! The recording can help you sleep better! Listening to the recording before bed helps your nervous system and body relax and prepare for sleep. And better sleep means less pain. The most noticeable benefit of getting good sleep is that your pain is lower the next day. Good sleep will also help you recover from surgery, illness, or injury. Use the recording to help you get to sleep, and use it again if you wake up in the middle of the night and need help falling back to sleep.

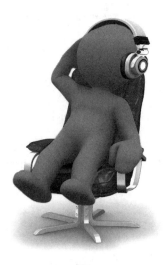

If you get in the habit of listening to the recording before bed and when you wake up in the night, just be sure to also listen to it sometime during the day so that you train your nervous system to be fully relaxed in the waking state as well as when you are in bed.

Can the recording help me take less pain medication?

Yes! The recording can help you reach your goal of taking less pain medication in several ways. First, you may have some anxiety or fear about taking fewer painkillers or less opioid medication. You may think, "If I take less medication, my pain will get worse." This is a common fear. In fact, most people who gradually taper their use of opioids—that is, who slowly take less and less opioids—discover they have *less pain*, even when they stop taking opioids completely.

To take fewer pills, try the following strategy:

1. Listen to the recording to lessen any anxiety or fears you may have about tapering opioids. When you begin to feel anxious about taking fewer pills, listen to the recording.

2. Once you begin tapering your opioid use, listen to the recording at least *twice daily*. This will calm you in the moment and will also *keep* your nervous system calm. It will help you stay more comfortable so you will need fewer painkillers.

What if I only have 5 or 10 minutes?

Use whatever time you have available and make the most of it. The first 5 minutes of the recording teach you diaphragmatic breathing. Again, diaphragmatic breathing is an important skill that slows your breathing *and* calms your nervous system. Know that you will gain some benefit even from listening to just a few minutes of the recording. Then see if you can work in a longer listening session later in the same day or the next day.

Beth's Tip: Even something small is better than nothing.

Take advantage of small breaks in your day to give yourself small doses of calming medicine. It only takes a few moments to slow your breathing and get into a pattern of diaphragmatic breathing. The first 5 minutes of the recording teaches you how to do this!

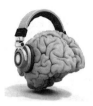

Calming My Nervous System

Date	Time	Before Relaxation Recording Stress Level	After Relaxation Recording Stress Level	Notes

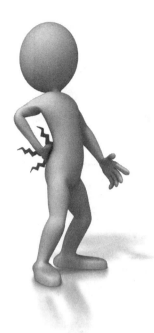

STEP 2
Understand Your Pain: It's More Than It Seems

You feel pain in your body, so it's natural to think of pain as simply a physical experience. But pain is more than just what you feel in your body—it's also what you feel emotionally.

The International Association for the Study of Pain (IASP) includes psychology in its definition of pain. The IASP defines pain as being a negative "sensory *and emotional experience.*"

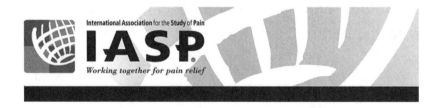

International Association for the Study of Pain

IASP.

Working together for pain relief

It may seem strange to consider that your experience of physical pain includes not just your body but also your emotions and your psychology.

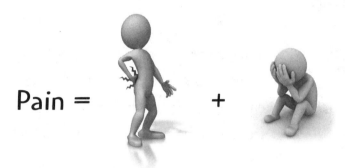

Pain =

+

Pain is a physical *and* a psychological experience.

Psychology is part of pain, but it is important to remember that:

❖ Your pain is NOT "all in your head."

❖ Your pain is NOT your fault.

❖ Your pain IS real.

Your pain IS real and it has a medical basis. Your nervous system plays a big role in your pain—no matter what kind of pain you have. Pain puts your nervous system on high alert, and in the long run this makes chronic pain worse. That's why it's so important to calm your nervous system for long-term pain relief, as you learned in Step 1: Quiet Your "Harm Alarm."

Your nervous system will also switch to high alert if you are often thinking negatively about pain and feeling anxious or worried about it. For this reason, it's important to understand and recognize when you are having the types of thoughts and feelings that put your nervous system on high alert. Then you can use skills to calm things down. By doing so, you will help yourself feel better emotionally and physically.

Treating Your Physical Pain AND Your Emotional Pain

While a lot of pain treatment only focuses on the physical part of pain, it's important to include psychological treatment in your pain care.

Imagine you have a car that is not working. After looking at the car, you learn that it is out of gas *and* it has a dead battery. In order for the car to drive, you need to have gas in the tank *and* a charged battery. Simply filling the car with gasoline will not be enough to make the car run. Both problems must be addressed before you will be on your way.

Beth's Tip: Knowledge is power.

Now that you understand that psychology is an important part of your pain, know that you can gain pain relief by learning skills that help you become aware of and gain control over your thoughts and feelings.

Similarly, overlooking the emotional part of pain leaves a big part of your pain untreated. Treating only the physical part of pain can mislead you into believing that you need more medication for relief. Often, the solution is not to take more medication; it's to treat your pain *differently* . . . and better. After all, if you only treat half of a problem, how can you be surprised when it doesn't work well?

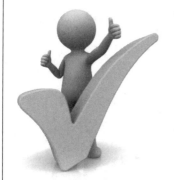

The second step in your opioid-free pain relief kit is understanding that psychology—how you think and feel—is an important part of your pain.

Your Emotions and Pain

Even though you "feel" pain in an area of your body, such as your back, all pain is processed in your nervous system. Your nervous system is your brain and spinal cord. Some of the areas of your brain that process pain also process your emotions, such as fear, worry, or feeling helpless. Your emotions and your pain are so closely related that they are "in the same neighborhood" in your brain.

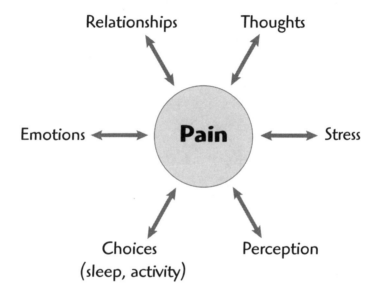

All pain is processed in your nervous system, which is made up of your brain and spinal cord. Everything that affects your nervous system also affects your pain. This includes your emotions, stress, expectations, beliefs, choices, and thoughts—your whole psychology!

21

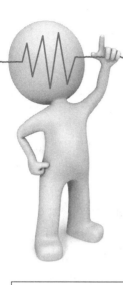

Harness the Hidden Power of Your Thoughts

In Step 2, we discussed how different factors, such as your emotions and stress, impact your pain. Now we will take it one step further.

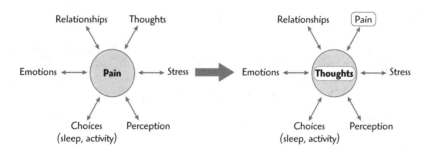

Every factor that impacts your pain
is related to your thoughts.

Relationships   Thoughts

Emotions ←→ **Pain** ←→ Stress

Choices   Perception
(sleep, activity)

Relationships   (Pain)

Emotions ←→ **Thoughts** ←→ Stress

Choices   Perception
(sleep, activity)

Your thoughts are so powerful that they can make your pain better or they can make your pain worse. In this section, we'll look at two examples that illustrate the power of thoughts to change pain for better or for worse.

An Example of How Thoughts Can Make Pain Worse

Marilyn's Story

I've had bad foot pain for about 5 years. It started with an injury and never got better. My pain is always there, and I find it hard to focus on anything else. Sometimes my pain flares beyond my normal pain. These are horrible episodes, and I find myself monitoring my pain a lot, to make sure I'm not beginning a bad flare. I definitely spend a lot of time thinking about my pain and worrying about it getting worse. It seems like there's nothing I can do about it except brace myself for a flare once I catch it starting.

Marilyn doesn't want to feel more pain—no one does. But she is stuck in a pattern of negative focus on her pain, and it is making her suffer more. She's dealing with a much steeper climb because of the way she is thinking and focusing on her pain.

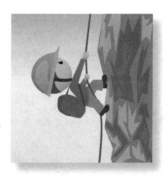

Beth's Tip: Remember, pain is your "Harm Alarm."

Now that you understand that psychology is an important part of your pain, know that you can gain pain relief by learning skills that help you become aware of and gain control over your thoughts and feelings.

It's important to gain control over negative thoughts about pain. Brain scan studies show that when your attention is focused on pain, pain grows in your brain—meaning that it actually gets worse. This happens because thinking negatively about pain lights up the same areas of the brain related to pain processing. **Your thoughts have the power to make your pain better or make it worse!**

Remember, all pain is located in your nervous system. With the right thoughts, you can calm your nervous system and lower your pain and distress. With the wrong thoughts (like Marilyn's), your "Harm Alarm" rings louder. Your pain gets worse when you focus on it. Focusing on pain often leads to something called *catastrophizing*. Catastrophizing is when you get in the habit of focusing on the fact that what's happening now is awful, and that the worst is yet to come (in other words, right now is a catastrophe, and you fear it will only get worse).

When you catastrophize, you cannot focus on anything but the pain and how awful it is, and you feel anxious worrying that the pain will get worse. Marilyn is catastrophizing when she keeps thinking a bad flare is about to happen. Catastrophizing is understandable, but it is important to recognize and treat it because it makes pain worse.

 Beth's Tip: Negative thoughts are part of your pain problem.

Negative thoughts make your "Harm Alarm" ring louder, which puts your nervous system on even higher alert and makes your pain worse.

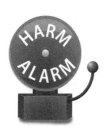 Your pain and distress increase as you catastophize and your nervous system goes on even higher alert. In this way, your nervous system works against you. The good news is you can learn mind-body skills and train your mind and nervous system to remain calm, thereby helping yourself have less pain. With the right information and skills, your nervous system will work *for* you.

> ***Beth's Tip:*** Calm thoughts are part of the solution.
>
> Calming thoughts soothe your "Harm Alarm" and calm your nervous system, lessen your distress, and reduce your pain.

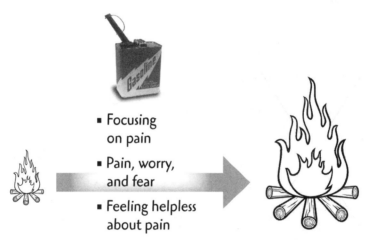

- Focusing on pain
- Pain, worry, and fear
- Feeling helpless about pain

Imagine this fire is your pain.

Negative thoughts and catastrophizing increase or "amplify" pain in your nervous system. It's like pouring gasoline on a fire!

Focusing on pain, catastrophizing and worrying about it, and feeling helpless about it work in your nervous system to worsen your pain. It's like pouring gasoline on the fire, making it grow larger.

The good news is that **you can learn to put the can of gasoline down and walk away from it, leaving negative thoughts behind.** Doing so will calm your nervous system, and reduce your pain and suffering.

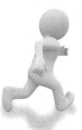

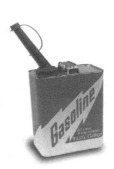

Taking Stock of Your Thoughts

Imagine that the fire in this illustration is your pain. Your thoughts either make the fire (your pain) better or worse. You can think of thoughts as adding either water or gasoline to the fire. Like water, positive thoughts reduce the fire and reduce your pain. Like gasoline, negative thoughts stoke the fire, making your pain grow larger.

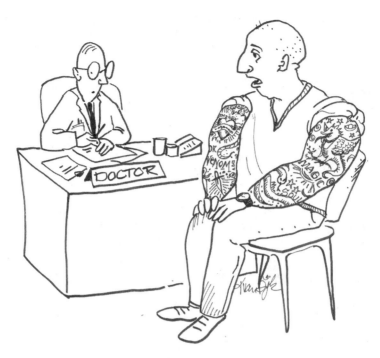

"I keep getting pins and needles in my arms."

It's important to understand whether your thoughts are working for you or against you—without you even knowing it!

Nobody wants more pain, but negative thoughts put your nervous system on high alert and make your "Harm Alarm" ring louder. Almost everyone has room for improvement when it comes to their thoughts about pain. Taking stock of your pain thoughts is the first move you can make toward gaining control of your pain.

Taking Stock of My Pain Thoughts

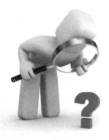

Consider the types of thoughts and feelings that you have when you are in pain. Listed below are 13 statements describing different thoughts and feelings that may be associated with pain. Using the scale,* indicate the degree to which you have these thoughts and feelings when you are experiencing pain.

	Not at all	To a slight degree	To a moderate degree	To a great degree	All the time
1. I worry all the time about whether the pain will end.	0	1	2	3	4
2. I feel I can't go on.	0	1	2	3	4
3. The pain is terrible and I think it's never going to get any better.	0	1	2	3	4
4. The pain is awful and I feel that it overwhelms me.	0	1	2	3	4
5. I feel I can't stand the pain anymore.	0	1	2	3	4
6. I become afraid that the pain will get worse.	0	1	2	3	4
7. I keep thinking of other painful events.	0	1	2	3	4
8. I anxiously want the pain to go away.	0	1	2	3	4
9. I can't seem to keep thoughts of pain out of my mind.	0	1	2	3	4

*The Pain Catastrophizing Scale (Michael Sullivan, PhD, et al., 1995) is reprinted with author permission.

	Not at all	To a slight degree	To a moderate degree	To a great degree	All the time
10. I keep thinking about how much it hurts.	0	1	2	3	4
11. I keep thinking about how badly I want the pain to stop.	0	1	2	3	4
12. There's nothing I can do to reduce the intensity of the pain	0	1	2	3	4
13. I wonder whether something serious may happen.	0	1	2	3	4

Now score it. Add your responses for all 13 items to get your total score. Your score will be between 0 and 52.

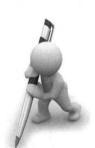

What Does Your Score Mean?

Your total score helps you understand whether your thoughts are working against you without you even knowing it! Knowledge is power, and knowing your score is your first step toward gaining control. Think of your total score as an opportunity to make some key changes that will help you feel better physically and emotionally. Research studies show that less catastrophizing equals less pain.

30–52: RED ZONE. Your score is high, but the good news is that as you reduce negative thoughts and mental focus, you will begin to feel a lot better. Your high score means that your brain is often focusing on pain and you tend to worry about pain a lot. But take heart: by regularly using the simple skills in this pain relief kit, you can reduce your score (and your pain!) quickly.

21–29: YELLOW ZONE. This is a common score range for people with chronic pain. By working to lower your score, you will have less pain and distress. Again, the good news is that the material in this pain relief kit will help you lower your score and feel better soon.

11–20: BLUE ZONE. Congratulations! Your score shows that you do pretty well at keeping yourself calm, even when you are in pain. By adopting some extra skills discussed in this book, you will soon find yourself scoring in the excellent zone.

0–10: EXCELLENT ZONE! You are a pain master and have excellent ability to keep your nervous system calm. You keep your mind focused on what you *can* do—and in doing so you help yourself feel better!

Now that you have a sense of where you are, let's look to where you want to go—***toward relief!***

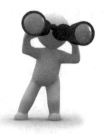

An Example of How Thoughts Can Make Pain Better

Luciana's Story

My neck pain began after a car accident. My pain is always there, but mostly it stays at a low level. In the beginning, I would get anxious about my pain, worry that it was only going to get worse, and immediately take a Vicodin to stop the whole cycle of pain and fear. Over the years, I've learned ways to help myself when my pain gets bad and I'm tempted to focus on the worst parts of it. Instead, I change my thoughts and steer them in a better direction. I remind myself that the pain flares come and go—this one will pass soon, too. I remind myself that there are several things I can do to help myself, including listening to my relaxation recording. I learned that if I keep my thoughts focused on pain, it only stresses me out and makes it worse. On the other hand, if I can focus on calming myself and also on changing my thoughts, I can change the way I feel. It may not take my pain away, but it keeps my pain low, and it definitely keeps me emotionally balanced. For me, that's half the battle, and it makes all the difference in the world.

Luciana still has chronic pain, but she has learned how to use the power of positive thoughts to keep her brain focused away from pain. Instead of pouring gasoline on her fire, she's sprinkling water on it. In other words, she keeps her nervous system focused away from pain, and in doing so she keeps her distress and pain low. She's helping herself feel better!

Perhaps most important, she doesn't feel at the mercy of her pain, or a victim of her life with pain. She's keeping focused on what she *can* do, and she's determined to make the best of it.

Positive thoughts are like giving yourself a helping hand. Imagine what you would say to your best friend if he or she were having a hard time with pain. Then use those same kind words to encourage yourself. Use the power of "best friend talk" to keep your nervous system calm.

Luciana's positive thoughts and mental focus

💧 Positive pain talk: "I always get through it" or "This too shall pass."

💧 Focus on what I can do to help myself feel better now.

💧 I talk to myself as if I were encouraging my best friend, Susan, with her pain. It's comforting and it works.

Luciana's pain

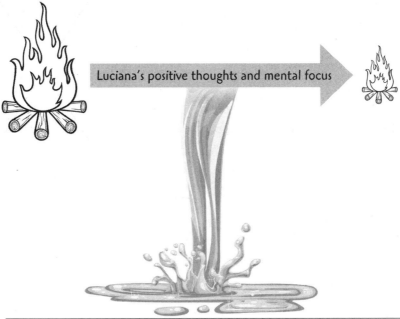

Luciana's positive thoughts and mental focus

> Positive thoughts are like sprinkling water on a fire. Positive thoughts calm your nervous system and help you feel better.

The examples of Luciana and Marilyn show how thinking positively and negatively leads to two different pain experiences—one better and one worse. Luciana experiences much less pain and distress than Marilyn because she knows how to keep her mind focused on thoughts that reduce her pain rather than making things worse with negative thoughts.

Now let's look at the example of Nico. Nico starts off like Marilyn, in a pattern of negative pain thoughts about his migraines, and turns things around to think more like Luciana. He learns to harness the hidden power of positive thoughts to feel better and gain control.

Nico's Migraine Challenge

When I feel a migraine coming on, I know it's going to be bad. I can't think of anything but how awful it is and how much I want it to stop! Right away I know it's only going to get worse over the next few hours. There's nothing I can do but take meds and wait it out.

Nico's Negative Thoughts and Mental Focus

 I feel a migraine starting and it's going to be bad.

 My migraine is awful and I want it to stop!

 It's only going to get worse.

 There's nothing I can do.

Nico is keeping his mind focused on how bad his pain is—and making his "Harm Alarm" ring louder as his nervous system goes on even *higher* alert.

Now, see what happens when Nico takes on his migraine challenge in a different way. Nico has created positive thoughts and calming statements to replace his old pattern of negative thinking that came up automatically when he felt a migraine coming on. In shifting his thoughts from negative to positive, he is calming his nervous system and quieting his "Harm Alarm."

Nico's Positive Thoughts and Calming Statements

THEN: Old Negative Thought	NOW: New Positive Thought and Calming Statement
I feel a migraine coming on and it's going to be bad.	I'm going to do what I can, right now, to help my pain stay as low as possible.
My migraine is awful and I want it to stop!	This migraine is a challenge—they always are. And they always pass. This one will pass, too.
It's only going to get worse.	I can help myself feel better by calming my mind and body. It won't take my migraine away, but it will ease my suffering.
There's nothing I can do.	I choose to focus on comforting myself right now when I need it most! I will listen to my relaxation recording, then fix some tea, dim the lights, and use my earplugs and eyeshade to create a soothing environment for myself.

Just like Nico, you can change your pain thought patterns and harness the power of positive thoughts to calm your nervous system and quiet your "Harm Alarm." Changing your thought patterns takes some practice. Even coming up with positive thoughts may seem strange at first. Like most things, if you practice regularly it will become easier. Over time, positive and calming thoughts will feel like second nature to you.

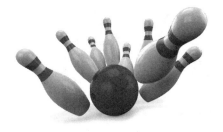

Make a game of it! Start noticing your thoughts—your self-talk—and make a game of coming up with positive statements to replace any negative thoughts you typically may have. Write your positive thoughts on flash cards, and have your cards handy so you can pull them out when you need them. Use *any* flash card to help interrupt the pattern of negative focus in your brain.

 Beth's Tips

Write positive thoughts and statements on flash cards.

Pull out a flash card when you hear yourself thinking negative thoughts. The card will interrupt the negative focus in your brain and will help redirect your negative thoughts toward relief.

Use the power of "best friend talk" to change pain.

As you notice your self-talk, ask yourself, "Would I say that to my best friend?" Oftentimes, the answer is "No!" Create positive statements—the supportive and kind statements that you would share with your best friend—and begin sharing them with yourself!

My Positive Thoughts and Calming Statements

OLD: My Negative Thoughts	NEW: My Positive Thoughts and Calming Statements

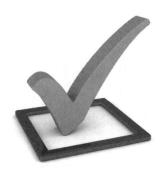

STEP 4
Pain Relief Actions
for Right Now

When you are in pain, or when you find yourself thinking negative thoughts and catastrophizing—*holding the can of gasoline!*—you can help yourself gain relief with soothing **pain relief actions.**

Pain relief actions are little things you can do to soothe yourself. Small, positive actions serve to stop catastrophizing. They direct you toward things you *can* do to help yourself in the moment. Making yourself feel pleasure, even if just for a brief time, interferes with your brain's pain circuitry. Little interruptions lead to big changes in pain over time—it's part of "rewiring" your brain away from pain. There is hidden power in doing something positive for yourself—even something small!

Taking Action to Feel Better

To feel better, it is important to have a list of simple, nurturing things you can do for yourself—almost like giving yourself a hug. Everyone craves comfort when in pain, and focusing on creating comfort is a great way to shift your focus away from pain. Steering your attention away from pain and focusing on something positive serves to calm your nervous system. It's like switching out gasoline for water to put out your fire, and it helps you feel better mentally and physically. Think of pain relief actions as good self-care—when you need it most! And remember that pleasure interferes with your brain's pain circuitry.

A Sample Pain Relief Action List

Here's an example of a general Pain Relief Action List to help soothe your mind and avoid catastrophizing:

1. Read positive affirmations.

2. Fix a cup of herbal tea.

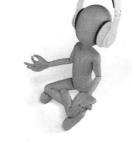

3. Review a gratitude list (5–10 things in your life that you feel grateful for).

4. Listen to the recording in this pain relief kit for 5 minutes.

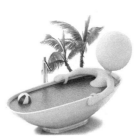

5. Check in with breathing; use the slow diaphragmatic breathing you learned on the pain relief recording for 5 minutes.

6. Go for a short walk alone or with a friend.

7. Sit in nature for 10 minutes.

8. Take a warm bath.

9. Call or text a supportive friend or loved one.

Your actions shape your brain activity and your nervous system, so be sure to do the things that will bring you support, comfort, and pleasure.

Create Your Pain Relief Action List

Create your personal Pain Relief Action List by jotting down a number of simple, soothing things you can do for yourself when you are struggling or in pain. Your list is just for you—it can be anything that brings you a bit of pleasure and positive focus in a moment of painful discomfort.

When you catch yourself catastrophizing or stuck in negative thoughts and feelings, pull out your list. Choose any item that will soothe you in the moment and point you toward relief.

 Beth's Tip: **Set yourself up for success.**

Create your Pain Relief Action List now so you have it ready and handy when you need it. Doing it now means you won't have to think or problem-solve when things are tough. Some days you may only need one pain relief action to lift you out of negativity. On other days, you may need several soothing actions. Be ready to take any action that will create a sense of calm nurturing. Feeling calm means that your nervous system is calm—and that's good pain medicine!

My Pain Relief Action List

1. _____

2. _____

3. _____

4. _____

5. _____

6. _____

7. _____

8. _____

9. _____

10. _____

11. _____

12. _____

13. _____

14. _____

15. _____

16. _____

17. _____

18. _____

19. _____

20. _____

Beth's Tip: Be gentle with yourself.

In addition to soothing you when you need it, your Pain Relief Action List fills another important role: it helps you learn to be gentle with yourself when you need it the most. Often, chronic pain can bring up unpleasant feelings of anger, disappointment, loss, and sadness. You may even feel anger at your body for having pain and for not being able to do some of the things you love. Be kind to yourself and help lessen your hurt feelings with your nurturing pain relief actions. Be compassionate with yourself and recognize that you—and your body—are doing your best. When you start to feel bad, take any soothing action right away. Doing so will move your energy in a positive direction as you help yourself feel better.

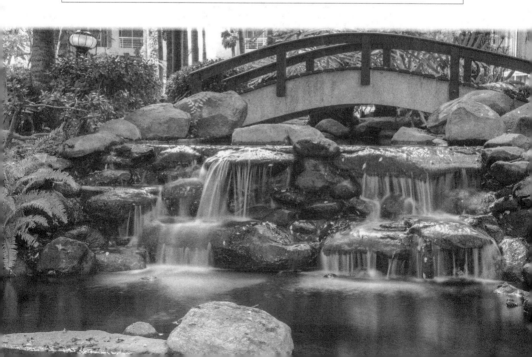

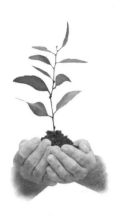

STEP 5
The Power of *Daily* Mind-Body Medicine

Your opioid-free pain relief kit will help you enjoy greater comfort with less pain medicine. Using the mind-body skills described in Steps 1 through 4 will help you reach your goal. Mind-body skills help you feel better. You can think of them as mind-body *medicine*! This type of medicine does not involve pills, however. Mind-body medicine is all of the things you do to keep your pain and distress low, such as calming your nervous system.

Many of the medicines doctors prescribe do not have full effect with the first pill. For example, medicine given for blood pressure, depression, or an infection must be taken for some time to have an effect. **Most medicines are taken daily, and they build up in your body over days and weeks before they work fully.**

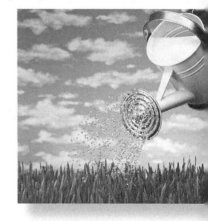

Even though mind-body medicine does not involve pills, it works similarly in that its effects grow over time. The more you do it, the better it works!

Each time you use your mind-body skills, it's like giving yourself a "dose" of mind-body medicine. It's like sprinkling a little water and sunshine on a seedling. The daily water and sunshine allow the roots to grow, anchoring the plant and making it stable. They also allow the stem to grow, giving the plant strength. Finally, the seedling blossoms into a full, leafy, mature plant. The daily water sprinkles and sunshine add up to big changes over time. The seedling grows stronger.

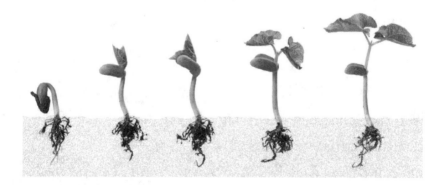

Mind-Body Medicine Works Best When You Use It Daily

Your daily practice of mind-body skills is like water and sunshine on the seedling— your results grow over time. Used daily, mind-body medicine keeps your pain and distress low. Research shows that mind-body medicine works to change, or "rewire," your nervous system. It helps your brain stop focusing on pain, your "Harm Alarm," negative thoughts—all of the things that put your nervous system on high alert and make your pain worse. Mind-body medicine puts you in the driver's seat as you steer your nervous system away from pain and toward comfort. Over time, your nervous system changes and your feelings of pain are reduced.

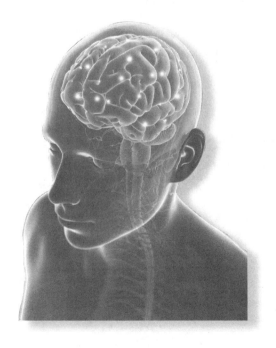

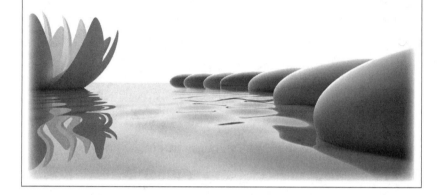

Keeping your nervous system calm is what gains you **lasting** relief!

Beth's Tip: Getting better takes time.

Be patient and remind yourself that the results of your daily calming will grow over the course of weeks. You will notice yourself feeling calmer almost right away, and that feeling will increase as you keep practicing your mind-body skills. Trust that the changes in your pain will unfold and grow over time. The first goal is to rewire your nervous system with daily practice. Pain changes are sure to follow soon!

Your Pain Relief Kit So Far

Let's review the key points in your opioid-free pain relief kit so far.

Step 1: Quiet Your "Harm Alarm"

Pain sets off your "Harm Alarm" and puts your nervous system on high alert. Having your nervous system on high alert makes you more sensitive to pain—and more sensitive to *everything*, including stress. In Step 1, you learned the importance of calming your nervous system to directly quiet the "Harm Alarm" and reduce your anxiety and pain.

Of course, quieting your "Harm Alarm" and calming your nervous system help you feel better in the moment—when your pain is bad or stress is high—but at first the effects might not be long lasting. You will feel better for a bit, and then your tension and pain will probably return to your normal daily level. That's expected.

Mind-Body Medicine

Occasional dose = A little bit of relief

Daily dose = Long-lasting relief

Calming your nervous system every day, however, helps your system rewire to an overall calmer state—with less pain, stress, and tension, and less need for pain medication. Daily calming leads to lasting comfort and relief.

Step 2: Understand Your Pain

Physical pain isn't just physical—it also includes your psychology. Psychology includes your emotions, thoughts, reactions, beliefs, stress, choices ... in other words, your everyday experience. In Step 2, you learned that tuning in to these factors every day will reveal opportunities for you to gain relief from pain.

Step 3: Harness the Hidden Power of Your Thoughts

You can't control all the events that happen in life. But one thing you *can* control is your *response* to those events. Recall from Step 3 that Marilyn and Luciana had two very different responses to their pain, and it made all the difference. Marilyn had negative thoughts and emotions—she focused on the worst parts of her pain and it made her suffer more. Negative thoughts and emotions lead to more pain, while positive thoughts soothe your mind and reduce suffering. Learning to put down the can of gasoline is important for containing the "flames" of your pain. Although you can't make your chronic pain go away entirely, feeling *less* pain because you don't respond as negatively to pain events— just like Luciana—is a very good thing!

Changing your pattern of thoughts works best with daily practice. After all, you are rewiring patterns in your brain. You have to train your brain how to think differently. Although it takes effort at first, over time, it becomes second nature. To harness the positive power of your thoughts, take stock every day.

Review your day and ask yourself:

❖ "Did I have any challenges with negative thinking today?"

❖ "How could I change my thinking about this challenge to help myself feel better?"

❖ "Can I 'step outside of myself' and view this situation differently?"

❖ "What would I tell my best friend if he or she were struggling with this same problem?"

Remember that the goal is to help yourself feel better. Notice how changing your thoughts allows you to feel calmer.

Using your Positive Thoughts and Calming Statements sheet (page 40) daily will make positive thinking second nature for you when handling pain and other life challenges.

Step 4: Pain Relief Actions for Right Now

Daily use of soothing pain relief actions will help your brain rewire faster. This is because every pain relief action serves to distract your brain from pain—it takes your focus away from your pain.

Each time you shift your focus away from pain and toward comfort, you are "shrinking" your pain experience. You are showing your brain how to suffer less.

Your pain relief actions (page 45) are powerful mind-body medicine when used regularly.

Step 5: The Power of Daily Mind-Body Medicine

As you just learned, Steps 3 and 4 work best when used daily—this is Step 5. It's the daily doses of mind-body medicine help you feel better overall, rather than just helping you get through a tough moment. Daily doses of mind-body medicine work by keeping your nervous system calm. It trains your brain away from pain!

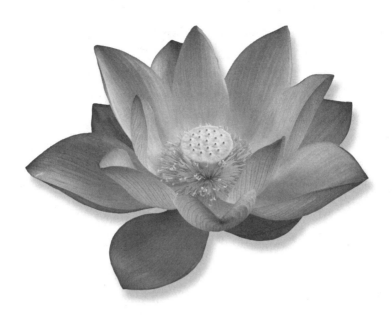

Used Daily, Pain Relief Actions Train Your Brain Away From Pain

Remember, your results build over time as your brain "learns" to be more comfortable and experience less pain and distress. When you are struggling with pain and distress, even something as small as fixing a cup of tea and taking five slow, deep breaths can be enough to break the cycle of despair. Breaking this cycle repeatedly weakens connections in your brain that are linked to pain and suffering.

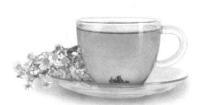

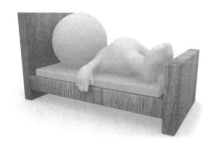

STEP 6
Sleep and Activity Are Pain Medicine

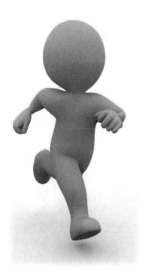

With chronic pain, it's common to have some trouble sleeping and being active. Pain can interfere with getting good rest. Pain can also get in the way of doing things you enjoy.

Maintaining a healthy balance of reasonable activity and good sleep is important because it helps keep your pain low. Let's take a look at why, and what you can do to improve both of these important parts of your pain relief plan!

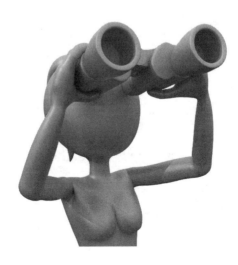

You know you feel better after a good night's rest. Here are some reasons why:

Sleep Is Good Medicine for Pain

❖ Sleep lowers inflammation in your body—it's an anti-inflammatory.

❖ Like food and water, you need sleep for survival. Humans cannot live without sleep.

❖ Without enough sleep, your body is under great stress. Stress makes your nervous system more sensitive to pain.

❖ Sleep helps your brain work better. Your memory is better and you can make better decisions about self-care when you get enough sleep.

❖ If you feel good mentally, you are more likely to do your mind-body exercises, and you will get better results.

❖ Sleep gives you energy the next day. You can use your energy to be more active and do the things you enjoy—things that keep your pain low.

❖ Research shows that sleep is one of the most important factors for lowering next-day pain. If you sleep well, your pain will be lower!

Opioids Are Not Good for Sleep

Although opioids may make you *feel* sleepy, they are not good for sleep! Opioids prevent you from reaching the deep stages of restorative sleep. If you are taking opioids now, a benefit of tapering down your use of them is that you will enjoy better quality of sleep once you are off opioids completely. If you have been taking opioids to help you get to sleep, talk to your doctor about melatonin, an over-the-counter supplement that is your body's own natural sleep hormone. Also be sure to listen to the recording included with this book right before bed to quiet your mind and prepare your body for sleep.

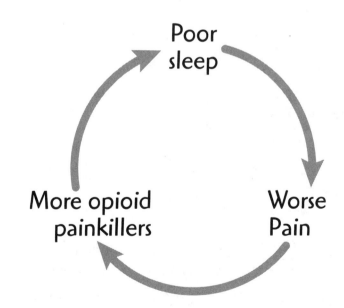

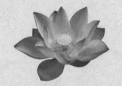

Beth's Tips for better sleep

Set a schedule. Think like a parent and set a regular sleep schedule for yourself. Children sleep best when they have a regular bedtime. Adults are no different. Pick a reasonable bedtime and stick to it.

Eat dinner early. Enjoy your final meal of the day a few hours before your bedtime. A full stomach can keep you up at night.

Dim the lights. Bright lights from lamps and electronic screens keep your brain alert, making it believe it's daytime, even though it may be late at night. Help your brain know that it's nighttime by keeping all lights low. Avoid lighted screens, such as TVs, computers, and cell phones, a full hour before bedtime. The blue light from these electronics is very powerful and can keep you up.

Make it quiet. Earplugs can create instant silence, allowing you to focus on your breathing and fall asleep fast. Earplugs also help you stay asleep because you don't notice sounds that might wake you up at night when you are wearing them. If disposable earplugs do not work for you, try custom-made earplugs. They are made of silicone and fit your ear perfectly. Talk to a local audiologist to find out options and pricing.

Prepare your mind and body for sleep. Listen to the recording that is part of this pain relief kit right before bed to calm your thoughts, slow your breathing, and lull your body and mind to sleep. If you wake up and have trouble falling back to sleep, listen to it again.

Avoid daytime sleep. To ensure you are tired and ready to sleep at bedtime, don't sleep during the day.

Avoid alcohol to sleep better. Alcohol may make you feel sleepy, but it actually disrupts your sleep, just like opioids do. Alcohol makes you sleep "light" and does not allow for deep, restorative sleep.

Avoid stimulants in the afternoon and night. Try avoiding caffeine after noon. Caffeine has long-lasting effects. Even drinking caffeine in the early afternoon can keep you up at night. Chocolate and sugar in the evening may also keep you awake, so try cutting them off earlier in the day and see if it helps you sleep better.

Nighttime is relax time! Relax before bed: take a warm bath, do some light reading, meditate ... anything that is relaxing to you. Avoid tackling major mental tasks right before bed, such as finances, problem solving, or thinking about anything stressful. Set an appointment with yourself to think about those things the next day.

Balance is key. With sleep, more isn't always better. It's possible to sleep too much, so finding a good balance is key. The goal is to feel good and be as active as possible the next day. Talk to your doctor if you are regularly spending most of the day in bed. It may be a sign of depression or another problem that your doctor can help you address.

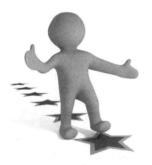

Activity as Pain Medicine

Like sleep, activity is great medicine for pain. Here are some reasons why a reasonable amount of exercise and activity helps you feel better:

❖ **Pain prevention.** Exercise and activity help you get stronger and prevent future pain that can arise if your body gets weak.

❖ **Strength.** Exercise and activity can reduce pain by strengthening muscles. For instance, you can gain relief from back pain by strengthening your core muscles.

❖ **Positive attitude.** Exercise and activity help keep your mind focused on positive actions—you are helping yourself get strong and feel better.

❖ **A reminder of what you CAN do.** Exercise and activity serve to remind you that you are able to do many things in spite of your pain. Instead of being sedentary and thinking about all the things you can't do, you are up and about and doing what you can.

❖ **Better sleep.** Exercise and activity help you sleep better at night, and that's good pain medicine.

❖ **Better brain chemistry.** Exercise and activity increase feel-good chemicals in your brain. These chemicals lower your pain and make you feel better.

❖ **Better mood.** Exercise and activity help you feel better in general, and they are proven treatments for depression.

Many people mistakenly believe that their pain must be reduced *before* they can become more active. In fact, it's often the other way around. Activity is a great way to reduce your pain!

Beth's Tip: Start where you are.

To become more active, the trick is to start where you are–not where you were, and not where you want to be. Many people fall into the trap of expecting themselves to be as active as they were before they had pain. It's not fair to expect yourself to be at that level, and trying to do so can cause you more pain. In short, it's a recipe to make you feel bad physically and emotionally.

Help yourself feel better by taking stock of how active you are right now. Be kind to yourself. It's OK if you are not very active now—small changes will add up to big differences over time.

Getting Started with Exercise

Talk with your doctor before beginning a new activity or exercise. Often, a physical therapy evaluation can help you learn which types of exercises are best for your pain—and which ones to avoid. And, a professional can help you determine an appropriate level of exercise, given your current fitness level.

How active am I?

Activity Type	Minutes per day (or distance)	Number of Days per week I engage in the activity
Walking		
Exercise/movement type*		
Household activity (such as housecleaning or yardwork)		

*List any different types of exercise or movements you are doing, such as gentle yoga, stretching, tai chi, water therapy, or physical therapy.

Set a SMALL Activity Goal

With activity goals, small is best. For one thing, small goals tend to be realistic. If your goal is realistic, you are more likely to achieve it, and you will be more successful. You want to feel better, and success feels good!

Set yourself up for success with the following steps:

1. **Pick a small, realistic activity goal.** Pick a goal based on your *current* activity level and ability. Avoid the trap of trying to start where you used to be and instead focus on where you are *today*. Doing so will set you up for success! Starting where you are is the first step toward reaching your goal.

2. **Rate your confidence.** After you pick a small, realistic goal, rate your confidence that you can complete the goal on a scale from 0 to 10, where 0 = no confidence and 10 = complete confidence.

Confidence Scale for Reaching My Goal

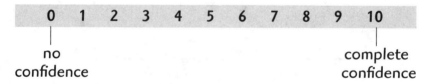

Consider Sally's Example

Sally's activity goal: Walk 3 days per week for 30 minutes on the track after work.

Sally's confidence rating. When Sally stops and thinks about it, she rates her confidence that she will reach her goal at 5 on the scale. She knows she's pretty tired after work and mainly wants to rest at that point. Her low confidence rating signals that she needs to revise her goal and make it easier for her to reach.

Sally's new goal: Walk 3 days per week for 15 minutes during the lunch hour at work.

Sally's new confidence rating. Sally knows she can do short walks at lunch on Mondays, Wednesdays, and Fridays when she does not have meetings. She changed her goal from 30 minutes to 15 minutes to make it more realistic. Also, she knows she's more likely to walk at work, especially if she asks Maria to go with her. With these changes she rates her confidence level at 8. She's pretty sure she can do this—and have fun doing it!

If you rate your confidence that you can reach your goal at 7 or less on the scale, make it a smaller goal that's within your reach. Small successes add up to big differences. Set yourself up for success with small activity goals that you know you can reach.

If you rate your confidence in being able to reach your activity goals at 7 or less, it just means you need to break up your goal into smaller pieces. Set yourself up for success with small activity goals that you can reach.

Remember, appropriate activity is great pain medicine. It keeps your mind and body healthy, strong, and flexible. You can take small steps and become more active over the course of weeks and months.

Example Activity Goal Sheet

Activity	How Much	Where and When	Confidence Rating, 0–10
Walking	15 minutes	Monday, Wednesday, Friday at noon at the park across from the office	8 - I can do this!
Gentle yoga	45 minutes	Saturday afternoon at the senior center	9 - Easy peasy.
Biking	30 minutes	Outdoors on Tuesday afternoons after work	5 - Not sure because weather may be bad.

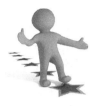

My Activity Goal Sheet

Activity	How Much	Where and When	Confidence Rating, 0–10

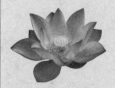

Beth's Tips for success with activity

Make it fun! You will be more active if it's fun. Walk with friends, take a gentle yoga class, join a warm-water aerobics class, take tai chi, or find a new neighborhood walking path. Social time and pleasure are good pain medicine—if you can make your activity pleasureable, it will be even stronger medicine!

Let technology motivate you! Try a gentle yoga or tai chi DVD that you can use right in your own home, or find a video on the Internet and follow along. A Fitbit or similar activity-tracking device can help you keep track of your daily steps and other fitness information and motivate you to meet your goals.

Deal with movement fear and anxiety. You can overcome fear and anxiety about movement by starting with very small goals. After all, the fear is that you will have more pain. The trick is to begin moving—slow and smart—so that you do not flare your pain (see Step 7: Preventing Pain Flares). Listen to your pain relief recording before exercise if you need to keep yourself calm so your pain doesn't increase. In the beginning, the goal isn't so much about making progress with activity—it's about reducing your fear about moving at all! As your distress lessens, you can consider a new activity goal—another very small step toward increased activity. Monitor distress and treat that first, but don't give up! Each time you achieve a small goal, you are overcoming your fear and anxiety—and success breeds more success.

If you find yourself stuck, work with a psychologist or mental health therapist who is skilled in treating pain-related fear. Don't let fear and anxiety stop you from moving forward with your goals. Get help and leave the suffering behind.

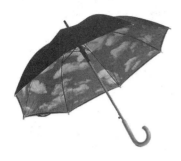

STEP 7
Preventing Pain Flares

Preventing pain flares is an important part of controlling your pain. **There's a lot you can do to prevent your pain from spiking and becoming worse.** Pain prevention is great medicine because when you prevent pain, you avoid suffering from more pain. Pain prevention strategies are positive actions that lower your pain.

Preventing Pain Flares: ACTIVITY

1. **Be Goldilocks.** Remember how Goldilocks needed porridge that was not too hot or too cold? She was looking for a temperature "sweet spot" for her porridge, a middle ground that was just right for her. Similarly with activity, you want to find a middle ground where you aren't doing too much or too little. Too much or too little activity will flare your pain and may lead to more medication use. To avoid having more pain, learn about good activity pacing.

2. **Pace yourself.** Good pacing means stopping *before* your pain flares. Be sure to stop activity when you still feel good—don't let feeling bad be your end point. If you feel bad, you went too far. In fact, a good activity goal is simply to practice good pacing.

Stopping when you feel good can be a challenge because it seems like you could be doing more. Remind yourself that good pacing will help you be *more* active in the days ahead, because you will not need downtime to recover from a pain flare.

Not only does good pacing help you be more active overall, it prevents the discomfort of the pain flare, *and* it prevents the dips in mood that come with pain flares. Pacing is great pain medicine. By pacing yourself, you can prevent many pain flares.

3. **Make small changes.** Good pacing also means making small increases in activity so you can allow your body to adjust before doing more. The goal is to succeed by slowly increasing your activity level over the course of weeks and months. Avoid the trap of trying to do too much too fast— there's a good chance that will lead you into a pain flare. By making small changes, you will prevent pain flares.

4. **It's OK to go slow!** Slow and steady wins this game. As is the case with many of the skills in this pain relief kit, consistency is the key. Consistent activity will gain you the best results and help prevent pain flares. It is better to walk a shorter distance a fews days each week than try to take a single very long walk on the weekend.

5. **Remember you are not alone.** Help yourself stay motivated by partnering with a buddy. Even if you cannot meet your buddy in person, you can call, e-mail, or text each other with progress updates and supportive messages. You can even find activity buddies online at websites and Twitter feeds for chronic pain support group.

Preventing Pain Flares: CALMING and SELF-CARE

Ultimately, everything in your opioid-free pain relief kit will help prevent your pain from flaring. Here are a few reminders from previous steps:

1. Keeping your stress and distress low calms your nervous system and focuses your brain away from pain. Listen to your pain relief recording regularly to prevent pain flares.

2. Using positive thoughts and statements focuses your brain away from pain. They also serve to keep you emotionally balanced so you make better choices about self-care. Good self-care helps prevent pain flares.

3. Soothing pain relief actions can help contain your pain from getting worse. If you find yourself in a flare, consult your Pain Relief Action List (page 45) and focus on soothing yourself.

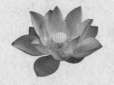 ### Beth's Tips for preventing pain flares

Know your warning signs. You are your own pain expert. You probably have a sense when your body and mind are reaching their limits. This may show up as mental, emotional, or physical fatigue. You may notice you become stressed and irritable—these are signs that your nervous system is taxed. Learn to be aware of your warning signs and take care of yourself before things get out of hand. Take frequent breaks during activity and throughout the day to check in with yourself and take stock of your needs. Calm your nervous system and assess how to best help yourself, and keep your pain in control.

Avoid pain "hangovers." You know the pain hangover well. It's when you do too much, overstress your body, and experience a pain flare. Remind yourself that pain hangovers are no fun and are not worth that little bit of extra activity. Pain hangovers contribute to low mood because they remind you of your limits in a negative way. It is much better to experience your physical limits by proactively deciding to hold yourself back as part of your feel-good self-care plan. It keeps you in control and feeling good mentally and physically.

When a flare strikes, learn from it. You will have another pain flare at some point. Use it as an opportunity to learn more about your pain. Was there anything you could have done to prevent the flare? Is there anything you can do differently in the future to have a different outcome? Avoid getting down on yourself if your pain flared because you overdid it. Instead, revise your activity goal and resolve to scale back so that going forward you are working within your body's limits to feel better. By doing so, you will be well on your way to preventing *future* pain flares.

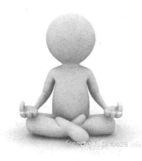

Step 8
Stress Relief = Pain Relief

Stress relief is an important part of your pain relief kit. Pain and stress are closely related—both put your nervous system on high alert!

Pain and stress are closely related—both put your nervous system on high alert.

Just like with pain, when you feel very stressed:

 Your muscles tense.

 Your breathing speeds up.

 Your heartbeat speeds up.

 Your blood vessels constrict.

 Fight-or-flight chemicals are released into your blood.

Chronic pain is stressful. Beyond the fact that it hurts, chronic pain can make it difficult to go about your daily activities and change your life. You may work less because of your pain, or maybe you cannot work at all, or you simply find it harder to get through your day.

The stresses related to chronic pain include the following and more:

- ❖ Financial problems

- ❖ Relationship issues

- ❖ Medical records and insurance concerns

- ❖ Managing medical appointments while dealing with other life responsibilities

As you have learned, pain causes mental stress, too. You may feel irritable when pain takes away your "stress buffer" or because you didn't sleep well due to pain. You may notice that when you are in pain, you are not your usual self, and that can be stressful, too. Even pain itself can be a sign of stress!

Common signs of chronic pain stress are:*

❖ Fatigue

❖ Irritability

❖ Muscle tension

❖ Anxiety and worry

❖ Feeling like you are not your usual self

❖ Withdrawing from friends and loved ones

❖ Feeling hassled by the world

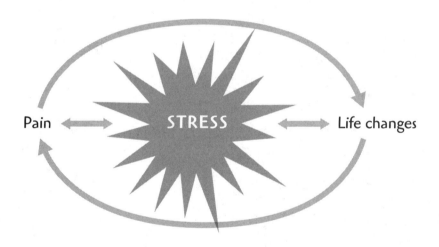

Pain ⟷ STRESS ⟷ Life changes

---

*Chronic pain can lead to more than just stress. It can also lead to ongoing depression or an anxiety disorder. If you have symptoms that are causing you a great deal of depression and distress, please talk to your doctor and ask about treatment options. You can get help for these issues.

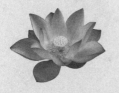

Beth's Tips for treating your stress and feeling better

Because stress causes the same changes in your nervous system as pain, you can treat stress the same way you treat pain—by calming your nervous system regularly.

Your Pain Relief Action List can be used to treat stress, too. Consult your Pain Relief Action List (page 45) to help yourself de-stress.

Make self-care your priority. It can be hard to put yourself first, but good pain management demands good self-care. Good self-care will ensure your physical and mental stress stays as low as possible. This means good sleep practices, good activity balance, good nutrition, and calming your nervous system daily.

Set limits. Be OK with saying no to others—and even to yourself. Sure you could drive your friend to the airport for her 10 p.m. flight, but doing so will disrupt your sleep schedule and set you up to be tired the next day—and be in more pain. Give yourself permission to say no so you can take excellent care of yourself. That way, you'll be feeling your best when you *do* see your friends.

Trust the wisdom of your body. Are you unsure whether you should or shouldn't do something? Close your eyes for a moment. Slow your breathing. Now, tune into your body as you consider your choices. See if you can observe tension or relaxation in your body as you consider one of your options. It may be a very slight twinge of tension or calm that you feel. Begin noticing the wisdom of your body, and go with the option that gives you the better feeling. Begin to think of relaxation as your own inner "Yes!"

Avoid stress traps. Alcohol and cigarettes are often mistakenly used as stress relievers. In fact, alcohol and cigarettes put more stress on your body and both lead to more pain over time.

Be active. Activity and exercise keep stress low. Use stress relief as a motivation to be active and stay on track with your exercise goals. Even small amounts of gentle exercise daily add up to big differences over time. Enlist a friend to take short walks with you—the buddy system is motivating and helps you stay on track.

Avoid stressful people and circumstances. Help yourself feel better by avoiding stress in your environment. Often you cannot eliminate stressful relationships, but you can find ways to spend less time with people who cause you stress. If you are having trouble avoiding stressful situations with other people in your life, consider working with a psychologist or therapist who can help you work on challenging relationships so they have less impact on you and your health. Look for opportunities to reduce stress in other areas of your life, too. Doing so is great pain medicine.

Ask for help. To reduce your stress burden, ask for help whenever possible. Ask for help taking groceries to your car. Ask your insurer if there is help available for understanding and filling out forms. Ask your clinic if they know of low-cost transportation services. Ask a friend to meet up and walk once a week. Start by asking questions to discover the help that is available to you.

Receive **help.** Once help is offered, be sure to accept it. Allow those who love you to contribute. Rather than rejecting the assistance others may offer you, practice receiving their kind gesture and gift of help. Graciously receiving these offers allows others to feel good about helping you!

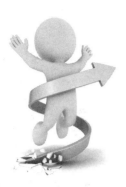

Step 9
Pleasure Is Pain Medicine

You just learned why less stress is good pain medicine. Similarly, pleasure is great medicine for pain! In fact, pleasure is the opposite of pain.

Pain   Pleasure

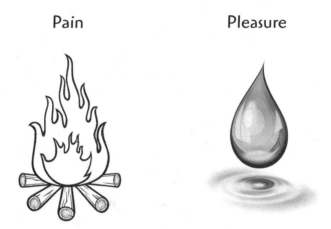

When you experience pleasure, it steers your brain away from pain. Your nervous system is also naturally calmed by pleasure, and this keeps pain low. In fact, the feel-good chemicals that are released in your brain during pleasure lower your pain and boost your mood.

Think of it like this: pain is physical and emotional in a negative way, and pleasure is physical and emotional in a positive way! Because pain and pleasure are opposites, focus on increasing your pleasure to shrink your pain.

Think of all the things that bring you pleasure, and create a pleasure list.

Here are some examples:

Time with friends

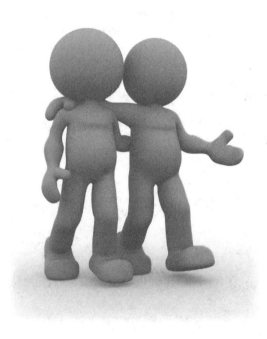

Time with family and loved ones

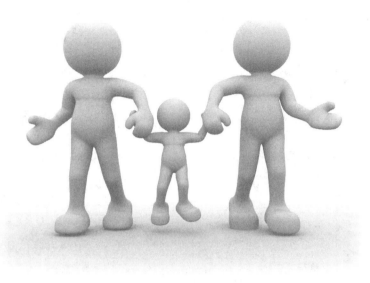

Intimacy

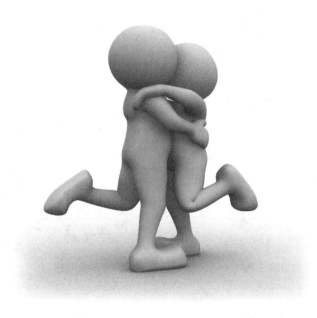

Hobbies

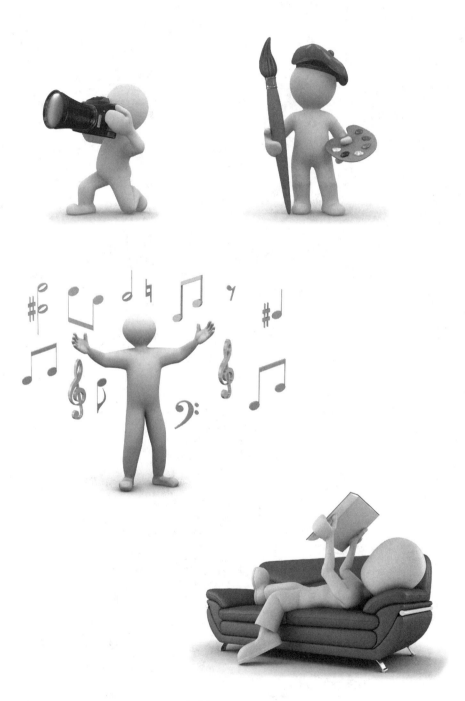

Beauty and nature

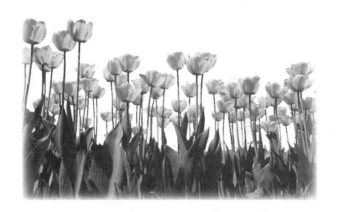

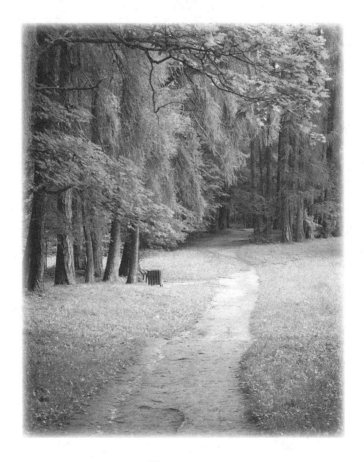

My Pleasure List

1. _____

2. _____

3. _____

4. _____

5. _____

6. _____

7. _____

8. _____

9. _____

10. _____

What brings you joy? Think about the things you can do right now that are enjoyable and meaningful to you. Maybe you cannot visit your brother in another state, but is calling him a possibility? Or maybe you cannot drive to the ocean today— but could you listen to an ocean sound CD while you relax? If you love the ocean, doing so will help you connect with it, and science shows that just the *memory* of things you love stimulates the same changes in your brain as the real thing!

Science shows that the pleasure of remembering the things you love stimulates the same changes in your brain as experiencing the real thing!

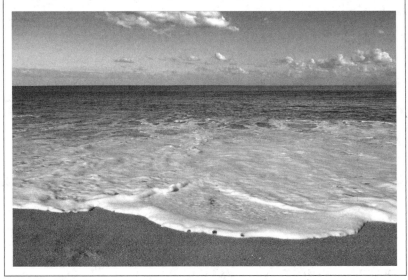

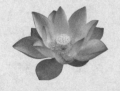

Beth's Tips for getting the most out of pleasure medicine

Daily doses work best! Giving yourself a daily dose of pleasure medicine will help counteract your pain. Set aside time for joy every day.

Treasure pleasure. Set aside time to really savor each moment of your pleasure activities. Noticing and appreciating the small details will boost your pleasure even more.

Shared pleasures can be wonderful. Spending time doing something pleasurable with someone you care about is double the fun and double the medicine. Even something as simple as giving another person a compliment is shared pleasure.

Keep it simple. Savoring a beautiful sunset, reading an uplifting poem or story, or walking around the block on a nice day are simple ways to experience pleasure right now. Look for simple ways to bring pleasure into your day without a lot of fuss or preparation.

The best pleasures are free. Have fun discovering free or low-cost pleasures. For example, having morning coffee in the sun or snuggling up with tea when it's raining outside are two examples of low-cost everyday pleasures. Bring awareness to the pleasure that is available to you each moment of every day.

Giving is receiving. Helping others is a great way to grow your *own* pleasure. Simple things such as offering directions or opening a door for another person are small gestures of kindness that bring you pleasure and a sense of connection to others. Look for small ways to give to people you know— or even to strangers—and watch your pleasure grow.

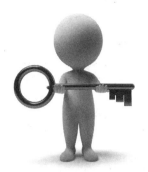

STEP 10

All Together Now: Your Complete Pain Relief Kit

Your key to success is taking everything you've learned so far—the previous nine steps to pain relief—and putting it all together. That is Step 10 in your opioid-free pain relief kit!

As you know, lasting relief comes from *living* all the steps in this kit and making them part of your daily routine. Putting together your complete pain relief kit may be easier than you think—and also fun. After all, everything in your relief kit focuses on helping yourself feel better—and that's something you've wanted for a really long time! It's exciting to think about feeling better and doing more of the things you enjoy and love.

Let's take a look at Alex's sample daily relief program. He provides a nice example of how to put all the steps in the kit into a complete program for lasting relief.

First, a little about Alex in his own words.

Alex's Story

I hurt my back in a car accident 5 years ago. It completely changed my life, and I never thought something like this would happen to me. I had to give up working for a year. Talk about stress . . . my medical problems were the least of it, too. How could I support my family when I was on disability?

I had three back surgeries, and my pain only got worse. It was devastating. All my hope built up and then each time: bam! I was taking a lot of opioid painkillers. They worked at first, then not so much over time. I kept needing more because my pain was bad. And I kept needing more because of the surgeries.

My sleep was terrible, I was frustrated and irritable, and my wife . . . well, all of this was testing our marriage. I felt like I had already lost so much and was at risk for losing it all. It got to where all I could see and feel was the pain. There was nothing good anymore. I felt like a failure as a husband and a man. I was depressed and it was only getting worse.

That's when my doctor and I talked and decided to do a slow wean off my opioids. I won't lie; I was scared at first. I thought, man, my pain is so bad now . . . what will it be like without the painkillers? I didn't think I could take it. It was a leap of faith, but I admit that I was so miserable I was willing to try anything, even if it sounded crazy. So I agreed to the slow wean. I mean, super slow. We took 6 months! My doctor said that there was no rush. After all, I'd been on them for 5 years. Why not take 6 months to ease the dose down comfortably? It made sense, and it helped me trust her plan.

We talked about how just taking away opioids wasn't going to suddenly make everything better. I needed a different kind of treatment—a plan to move forward and create my own relief. That's when she turned me on to this program. I threw myself into it because, well, it was the alternative and I was determined to make it work. I'm super motivated because I want to be better for my family. They deserve it, and I deserve it, too. I just hadn't known there was so much I could do to help myself . . . so I focused on the pills instead.

Here's the thing: I went down on my opioid dose and had a big surprise. Instead of my pain getting worse, it got better. Not a lot better, but better. For me, just that was huge! It showed me that the so-called "painkillers" weren't doing as much as I thought they were . . . so why take them? I learned that with the right medical plan, I could stop the pills and avoid the side effects—without being overwhelmed by pain like I had feared I would. In fact, my thinking got clearer, my mood was better, and I started sleeping like I used to. I began waking up feeling good again.

Now, every day, my pain relief is my number one priority. Because if I have less pain, I have a better life. If I have less pain, I have a better marriage. If I have less pain, I can focus on why I'm even here and what I want to do with my life. My energy is freed up. I feel powerful now, and that's a new feeling! For 5 years I felt I had no power, and it was awful. So, you bet, I focus on this like my life depends on it. Because one thing is for sure—my *quality* of life does depend on it!

Alex's Daily Program

Each day, Alex fills in his Complete Relief Plan—entering information on what he did that day. He also sets his activity and sleep goals for the next day. Having a clear plan for the day helps him stay focused and meet his goal.

Date	Calming My Nervous System	Positive Thoughts & Soothing Actions
5/1	Relaxation: 11 am, 8 pm. Breathing: Listened to the first 5 min of the relaxation recording at 9 am and the whole thing at bedtime.	Felt back pain coming on and began to focus on it and worry about it ruining my Sunday. Went right into my Soothing Actions and did 3 of them! Then pulled out 2 positive flashcards to get my head out of the thinking "danger zone."

Activity Goal	Sleep Goal	Pleasure Medicine
Goal: Walking 20 min What Happened Today: The day got away from me but I did get a solid 10 min walk in with Julie. Housework too.	Goals: Get to bed by 10 pm. No phone or computer after 9 pm. What Happened: No phone/computer after 8 pm! In bed at 10:30. Not always hitting goal but I'm more mindful. Getting there. May revise my bedtime goal to 10:15 pm.	Ate burgers with Julie on the balcony and watched the sunset. Felt really grateful. Spent time with Julie talking about what was going well—focusing on the positive and giving the good feelings room to grow!!

Now put together your own Complete Relief Plan:

Date	Calming My Nervous System	Positive Thoughts & Soothing Actions

Activity Goal	Sleep Goal	Pleasure Medicine

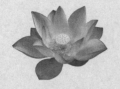

Beth's Tips for Succeeding with Your Complete Relief Plan

Write it out. You may be tempted to just read over the plans and put it together in your mind rather than on paper. Take a moment and actually write out your Complete Relief Plan. Research shows we learn best by writing. If you write down your plan, you will have it clear in your mind and will remember it later on. These are keys to following through and reaching your goals.

Plan ahead. Your Complete Relief Plan isn't just a record of what you are doing—it's your plan for continual success. Each evening, fill out your activity goals and sleep goals for the next day. That way, you have a plan mapped out and you are prepared.

Pay attention and revise as needed. Notice what's working and what's not working. If you see yourself falling short of a goal, don't worry. Falling short just means that you probably need to revise that goal. Make your goals more realistic, and make sure you are confident you can achieve each goal you set. Doing that means you are setting yourself up for success.

Be flexible. Life can get in the way of our goals, and being flexible helps. What seemed realistic on Monday may not be realistic on Thursday after you come down with a cold. Give yourself permission to be flexible and adjust for daily life changes. Revise your goals with what's realistic for you each day, given your current circumstances.

Celebrate your wins. Choose to focus on what's going well, and consult your list of positive thoughts and calming statements as needed. If you find yourself not following your daily plan, resolve to simply begin again with your Complete Relief Plan. Recommitting to a new daily plan is a big win and something to celebrate in and of itself. It's your first step to feeling better.

Every little bit counts. Remember that the goal is to take small steps forward. Making small changes each day adds up to big differences over time. You are more likely to stick with the small daily changes because they are doable and realistic for you, and small changes easily become part of your new routine. Each time you calm your nervous system, each time you have a positive thought, and each time you take a soothing action, you are helping train your nervous system away from pain.

Your Complete Relief Plan puts you in charge of your nervous system and how you feel.

Remember that your daily program works to train your brain away from pain. Daily practice gives you relief and a richer, more pleasurable life!

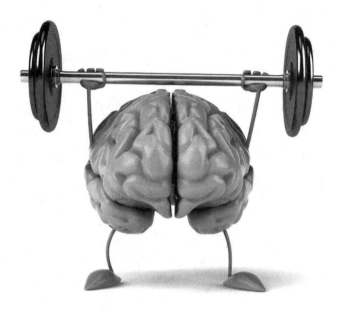

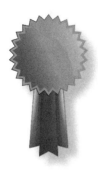

CONGRATULATIONS!

You now have the information and skills you need for opioid-free pain relief. Have fun making the complete pain relief kit part of your daily life, and enjoy the results of your effort.

Sometimes, extra support can be helpful, even necessary. If you find yourself having trouble getting on track or staying on track with your relief kit, it may be a sign that you can benefit from extra support. Consider working with a health psychologist, a pain psychologist, or a mental health professional skilled in pain management. Think of them as your pain relief coaches. Share this book with your therapist and talk about your goals and your barriers. Meeting with a therapist every week or two may give you the structure and extra motivation to get over any speed bumps that are holding you back. Ask your doctor for advice if you are unsure about how to locate a good therapist.

Finally, reading this book more than once can really help. You will discover bits of information that you missed the first go-around! And, reading it again will give your brain a chance to absorb and learn all of the information.

Happy reading!

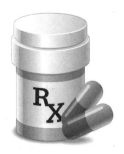

Opioid Medications: What You Need to Know

What Is Opioid Pain Medication?

Some types of pain medication can be purchased over the counter in any pharmacy and even many grocery stores. Over-the-counter nonprescription pain medications include Tylenol (acetaminophen), Advil (ibuprofen), Aleve (naproxen), and ordinary aspirin. Other pain medications require a prescription from a doctor or nurse. Opioids are a class of pain medication that requires a prescription.*

Common Opioid Medications and Brand Names

❖ acetaminophen/hydrocodone (Vicodin, Norco)

❖ acetaminophen/oxycodone (Percocet)

❖ oxycodone (Oxycontin, Roxicodone)

❖ oxymorphone (Opana)

❖ fentanyl (Duragesic, Abstral)

❖ hydromorphone (Dilaudid, Exalgo)

---

*Opioids are most often prescribed in pill form or as skin patches.

Opioids for Short-Term Pain

In many cases, the pain from injuries (and even surgery) can be helped with over-the-counter medications alone. A doctor or other qualified health care provider may also prescribe opioids for this type of pain. When opioids are prescribed for brief pain, which is sometimes called *acute pain*, the opioids are stopped once healing begins and pain stops.

Opioids for Chronic Pain

State and national guidelines now recommend limiting use of opioids. In general, it's good to avoid taking opioids for chronic pain. For one thing, unlike the short-term pain that occurs after an injury, chronic pain has no clear end. Before the new recommendations, physicians used to hand out opioid prescriptions that continued for years. Long-term opioid use is linked to many side effects and problems, including:

* Poor sleep
* Poor mood
* Low testosterone
* Low estrogen
* Increased pain
* Fatigue
* Constipation*

---

*For more information about specific opioid risks, see *Less Pain, Fewer Pills: Avoid the Dangers of Prescription Opioids and Gain Control Over Chronic Pain* by Beth Darnall, PhD (Boulder, Colo.: Bull Publishing, 2014).

An even bigger problem with opioids is that these side effects cause *more pain*. For instance, while opioids may make you feel sleepy at night, they actually cause sleep problems. Opioids stop you from reaching the deep stages of sleep that help you feel rested in the morning. When you don't sleep well, next-day fatigue causes more pain—leading to more medication use. You can see how opioids can lead to bad cycles of more pain and more pills. It's a slippery slope!

Even though opioids are taken to decrease your pain, they can also increase your pain by causing you to be more sensitive to pain throughout your body. Taking more opioids does not help this problem. The solution is to stop the opioids and treat the pain differently.

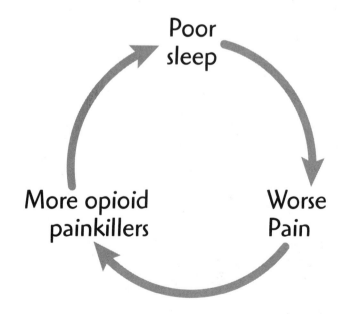

Opioids: A Slippery Slope
Using Opioids for More Than Just Treating Physical Pain

As you have learned, opioids change many things besides your pain, such as your sleep patterns and hormones. Opioids can also change your mood and feelings. These 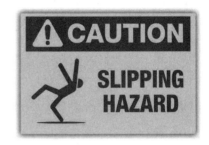 powerful drugs can cause a pleasant experience, or a "high," which is why there is an illegal market for opioids as narcotic street drugs. This is one reason why opioids are controlled substances that are monitored in the United States by the US Drug Enforcement Administration (DEA).

Opioids Carry Risks for Overuse and Addiction

When prescribed for chronic pain, opioids carry risks for overuse and addiction. Many people mistakenly believe that if a medication is prescribed by their doctor, then it is safe and without risk. **In fact, it's possible to have problems with opioids** *even when taking them exactly as prescribed.* It can be a slippery slope because opioids can make you feel better in the short run—physically and also emotionally.

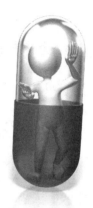

It's common to worry about pain, and even to have some fear about pain. Opioids can relieve fear and worry and lead you to feel better temporarily—but it's another slippery slope. Physical pain and emotional pain are very closely related. It is easy to begin taking opioids for a physical problem but end up taking more to treat the emotional aspects of your condition. It's also easy to remain on opioids for a long period of time because they seem to relieve stress and unpleasant emotions.

This book teaches you ways to calm your own worry and fear about pain and gain relief *without* opioids. The use of this opioid-free pain relief kit has little or no health risks, thereby keeping you safe and off the slippery slope. It means *you* are in control—not the pill bottle!

Reading this book is a testament to your desire to help yourself. Congratulations for learning the 10 steps to gain relief from chronic pain—you are well on your way. Sticking with your plan will gain you the comfort and control you desire, and the better quality of life you deserve.

You *can* do this!
Stick with the plan—and good luck!

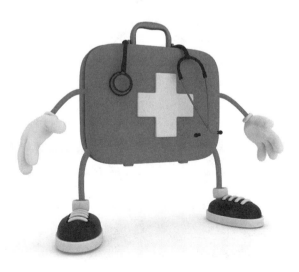

Resources

For articles, videos, and a blog by author Beth Darnall, visit www.bethdarnall.com. Her website contains two recommended pain psychology videos, both available at:

http://bethdarnall.com/videos

"Unlocking the Medicine Box in Your Mind" (short version, 37 minutes)

"Opening the Medicine Box in Your Mind" (long version, about 60 minutes)

Dr. Darnall also writes the *Less Pain, Fewer Pills* blog for *Psychology Today*, where she offers additional tips for pain relief and more information on pain psychology. Visit the blog at www.psychologytoday.com/blog/less-pain-fewer-pills.

Dr. Darnall recommends the following books for readers in search of in-depth information about chronic pain, chronic pain management, and alternatives to opioids:

Less Pain, Fewer Pills: Avoid the Dangers of Prescription Opioids and Gain Control Over Chronic Pain by Beth Darnall, PhD (Boulder, Colo.: Bull Publishing, 2014, 2016).

Living a Healthy Life with Chronic Pain by Sandra LeFort, MN, PhD, Lisa Webster, RN, Kate Lorig, DrPH, Halsted Holman, MD, David Sobel, MD, MPH, Diana Laurent, MPH, Virginia González, MPH, and Marian Minor, RPT, PhD (Boulder, Colorado.: Bull Publishing, 2015).

About the Author

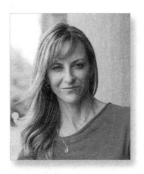 **Beth Darnall, PhD,** is clinical associate professor at Stanford University School of Medicine in the Department of Anesthesia, Perioperative and Pain Medicine. A clinical psychologist, she has treated chronic pain exclusively for the past 15 years, and lived through her own chronic pain experience. She currently treats patients individually and in groups at the Stanford Pain Management Center. She is a pain scientist at the Stanford Systems Neuroscience and Pain Lab whose research is funded by the National Institutes of Health. Her work broadly focuses on empowering people living with chronic pain by expanding access to low-cost, high-quality pain care that emphasizes pain psychology skills. She has been interviewed by *MORE Magazine, Women's Health, Men's Health, Healthline,* the *National Pain Report* and *ABC News.* Please visit www.bethdarnall.com and follow her on Twitter @bethdarnall.

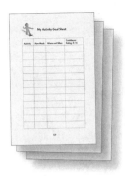

Worksheets

The following pages contain 3 extra copies of the worksheets introduced in this book.

❖ Calming My Nervous System

❖ My Positive Thoughts and Calming Statements

❖ My Pain Relief Action List

❖ My Activity Goal Sheet

❖ My Pleasure List

❖ My Complete Pain Relief Kit

As you continue to work your pain relief plan, you can use the new sheets to update your goals, lists and plans to reflect where you are right now. Focusing on where you are right now will help you create appropriate new goals and actions that will help get you where you want to be.

You may also download copies of these PDF forms at:

www.bullpub.com/downloads

Remember that you have support to help you gain relief. You now have the tools and the structure in place to help yourself feel better.

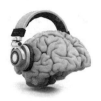 # Calming My Nervous System

Date	Time	Before Relaxation Recording Stress Level	After Relaxation Recording Stress Level	Notes

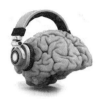

Calming My Nervous System

Date	Time	Before Relaxation Recording Stress Level	After Relaxation Recording Stress Level	Notes

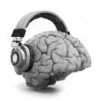 # Calming My Nervous System

Date	Time	Before Relaxation Recording Stress Level	After Relaxation Recording Stress Level	Notes

My Positive Thoughts and Calming Statements

OLD: My Negative Thoughts	NEW: My Positive Thoughts and Calming Statements

My Positive Thoughts and Calming Statements

OLD: My Negative Thoughts	NEW: My Positive Thoughts and Calming Statements

My Positive Thoughts and Calming Statements

OLD: My Negative Thoughts	NEW: My Positive Thoughts and Calming Statements

My Pain Relief Action List

1. _____

2. _____

3. _____

4. _____

5. _____

6. _____

7. _____

8. _____

9. _____

10. _____

11. _____

12. _____

13. _____

14. _____

15. _____

16. _____

17. _____

18. _____

19. _____

20. _____

My Pain Relief Action List

1. _____
2. _____
3. _____
4. _____
5. _____
6. _____
7. _____
8. _____
9. _____
10. _____
11. _____
12. _____
13. _____
14. _____
15. _____
16. _____
17. _____
18. _____
19. _____
20. _____

My Pain Relief Action List

1. _____
2. _____
3. _____
4. _____
5. _____
6. _____
7. _____
8. _____
9. _____
10. _____
11. _____
12. _____
13. _____
14. _____
15. _____
16. _____
17. _____
18. _____
19. _____
20. _____

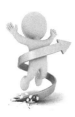

My Activity Goal Sheet

Activity	How Much	Where and When	Confidence Rating, 0–10

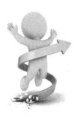

My Activity Goal Sheet

Activity	How Much	Where and When	Confidence Rating, 0–10

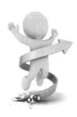

My Activity Goal Sheet

Activity	How Much	Where and When	Confidence Rating, 0–10

My Complete Relief Plan

Date	Calming My Nervous System	Positive Thoughts & Soothing Actions

Activity Goal	Sleep Goal	Pleasure Medicine

My Complete Relief Plan

Date	Calming My Nervous System	Positive Thoughts & Soothing Actions

Activity Goal	Sleep Goal	Pleasure Medicine

My Complete Relief Plan

Date	Calming My Nervous System	Positive Thoughts & Soothing Actions

Activity Goal	Sleep Goal	Pleasure Medicine

My Pleasure List

1. _____

2. _____

3. _____

4. _____

5. _____

6. _____

7. _____

8. _____

9. _____

10. _____

My Pleasure List

1. _____

2. _____

3. _____

4. _____

5. _____

6. _____

7. _____

8. _____

9. _____

10. _____

My Pleasure List

1. _____

2. _____

3. _____

4. _____

5. _____

6. _____

7. _____

8. _____

9. _____

10. _____

Index

Note: Page numbers in italics indicate worksheets.

headphones, 8
help
  asking for, 84
  receiving, 84
hobbies, 88
hydrocodone, 107
hydromorphone, 107

I

International Association for the
  Study of Pain (IASP), 17
intimacy, 87

J
joy, 91

M

memories, 91
mind-body skills, 47–55
Mobic, 107
movement fear and anxiety, 70–71
My Activity Goal Sheet worksheet,
  69
My Pain Relief Action List
  worksheet, 45
My Pleasure List worksheet, 90
My Thoughts and Calming
  Statements worksheet, 40

N

nature, 89
nervous system, 1–6
  quieting, 5–6
Norco, 107

O

Opana, 107
opioids
  avoiding use of, 113
  common medications and brand
    names, 107
  definition of, 107
  increased pain caused by, 110
  risks for overuse and addiction, 112
  for short-term pain, 107
  side effects, 109–110
  sleep and, 59, 110
  slippery slope of, 111–112
  what you need to know, 107–113
overuse of opioids, 112
oxycodone, 107
Oxycontin, 107
oxymorphone, 107

P

pacing yourself, 73–75
pain
  acute, 108
  chronic, 1, 109
  definition of, 17–18
  emotions and, 21
  as "Harm Alarm," 1–6
  as physical and psychological
    experience, 17–21, 52
  understanding, 17
pain flares
calming, 76
learning from, 78
Pain Relief Action List and, 76
preventing, 73–78
self-care, 76

Your *Enhanced Pain Management: Binaural Relaxation Audio file* is located here:

www.bullpub.com/catalog/EPM

The Publisher grants to purchasers of *The Opioid-Free Pain Relief Kit* permission to stream the audio file titled *Enhanced Pain Management: Binaural Relaxation*, by Beth Darnall, PhD.

This license is for personal use only and does not grant purchasers the right to reproduce or share *Enhanced Pain Management: Binaural Relaxation* in any form under any circumstances.

Customers who would like to purchase a CD version of *Enhanced Pain Management: Binaural Relaxation* can order copies at www.bullpub.com/catalog/EPM